WHAT IS TINNITUS?

T innitus is the perception of a sound not caused by an outside source. This condition affects millions of people and can be extremely disruptive to one's life, especially if it leads to feelings of depression and anxiety.

Other individuals cannot hear tinnitus itself, and only the individual who has this condition will perceive the sounds that go along with it, such as buzzing or hissing noises.

Different types of sounds heard

People who have tinnitus often hear various sounds in their ears, such as:

- Hissing

- Ringing/buzzing

- Roaring/thundering

- Clicking

- High-pitched whistling

However, each person experiences these symptoms differently and may hear different sounds depending on the severity and length of time they experience this condition.

People affected by tinnitus

As mentioned previously, about 25 million Americans have tinnitus (Chair & Limb, 2018). However, many people do not report experiencing tinnitus because they have become accustomed to the noise or have learned to manage it as part of their everyday lives.

There are risk factors that may heighten the chances of developing tinnitus. Here are a couple of factors:

• Being exposed to loud noises for extended periods, like those who listen to music through headphones or attend concerts. It is highly prevalent among individuals above the age of 50. When necessary, not wearing hearing protection can cause damage over time that may lead to this condition.

• Have a family history of tinnitus since it seems genetic in many cases. Suffering from certain medical conditions, including heart disease and high blood pressure that could affect circulation throughout the body, including the ears, can contribute to experiencing this condition. Being stressed out or tired because these examples drop the brain's ability to cope with auditory information properly.

Causes

Unfortunately, the exact cause of tinnitus is not fully understood by researchers and medical professionals. However, they do believe that several factors contribute to its development, including:

• **Loud noises**

Prolonged exposure to loud noises above 80 decibels can result in nerve damage, leading to tinnitus symptoms. This often occurs when individuals work in a factory or other occupation involving frequent exposure to excessive noise levels. Hearing loss due to aging or other health conditions such as Meniere's disease can also risk developing Tinnitus. These issues compromise one's ability to hear properly, leading to heightened sensitivity causing the brain to perceive sounds where none exist.

• **Injury**

There have been reports of patients experiencing intense tinnitus symptoms after a head injury, which has been linked to the development of this condition in some cases.

• Medication

In some instances, certain medications can cause an individual to experience ringing or buzzing sounds in their ears associated with Tinnitus. This can occur when these drugs interfere with serotonin and dopamine levels, affecting how a person processes sound signals in the brain.

• Certain health conditions

Individuals who have problems with blood flow in their body, such as those who have heart disease or high blood pressure, tend to report more experiences with Tinnitus because vascular issues inhibit circulation throughout the body, including the ears. Meniere's disease also involves excessive fluid retention in one's inner ear, leading to tinnitus symptoms.

• Earwax

Excessive buildup of earwax may also contribute to tinnitus. It creates an unwanted blockage in the ear and reduces hearing, which increases a person's likelihood of experiencing this condition.

Types

Tinnitus has types and subtypes. Here are as follows:

• **Primary Tinnitus** - This occurs when your tinnitus is not caused by another medical condition such as an ear injury or a tumor.

• **Secondary Tinnitus** - Here, tinnitus results from another health issue that needs treatment, such as certain neurological conditions (i.e., multiple sclerosis) and weakened bones in the skull as a side effect of taking certain medications. If you believe your case of Tinnitus may be due to any of these causes, then speak with your doctor about it and discuss whether or not you ought to see an audiologist for further testing and sound therapy.

• **Subjective Tinnitus** - This is considered the most common type, mainly caused by exposure to extremely loud noise. Often, this type of tinnitus varies with the intensity and length of the noise. People with this type of condition tend to struggle with other sounds in their surroundings, making it hard to focus on the most important sounds. The good news is that hearing aids distract from the ringing or buzzing sound caused by this condition so that you can focus on the most important sounds in your environment.

• **Sensory Tinnitus** - This is a form of subjective tinnitus whose cause remains unknown. However, it is typically considered a side effect of an impaired auditory system. With a well-established tinnitus management program, its negative effects are significantly reduced. People with this condition tend to experience an off-balance.

• **Somatic Tinnitus** - This condition is closely related to one's physical movement and touch. It is also referred to as conductive tinnitus, which is caused by external functions rather than just neurological problems. If you have a muscle spasm around your neck or ear, the chances are you will develop somatic Tinnitus. Other mechanical sources like a pillow that causes the neck to twist or dental problems are potential sources of somatic Tinnitus. To treat somatic Tinnitus, you can use sound therapy or massage therapy.

• **Objective Tinnitus** - This is a very rare type of Tinnitus; but is also the only type that others can hear, usually utilizing a stethoscope. Often, it is known to move in tandem with one's heartbeat.

TREATMENT OPTIONS FOR TINNITUS

T innitus can have a very negative impact on one's life, especially if it leads to feelings of depression, anxiety, and in some cases, even suicide. If your tinnitus causes you to experience any of these symptoms, you must discuss them with your doctor so you can be treated accordingly.

There are various treatment options for people who suffer from tinnitus, including sound therapy, medications, mindfulness practices, cognitive behavioral therapy (CBT), and lifestyle changes.

Sound Therapy

There are two main types of sound therapy for this condition: masking devices or hearing aids to cover up the sounds that you hear associated with Tinnitus. Using these devices makes it possible to create sounds that block out the noise that may be irritating you and causing stress. Some examples of these devices include White noise generators: These produce a constant sound that can mask the annoying sounds you hear associated with Tinnitus. Electronic sound generators: They produce computerized sounds so patients can choose between various settings and frequencies to find something that works for them.

Pros: Sound therapy offers sufferers an effective means of reducing stress associated with Tinnitus in many instances. It is also relatively inexpensive compared to other options out there for this condition.

Cons: The use of sound generators can be bothersome or irritating for some people who suffer from tinnitus symptoms. Therefore, it is important to learn how best to adjust the frequency and volume accordingly, positively impacting your symptoms while allowing you to continue doing what needs to be done throughout each day.

Cognitive Behavioral Therapy (CBT)

This type of therapy has been found to provide relief from the effects of chronic Tinnitus for many individuals who suffer from this condition by teaching them strategies to deal with stress, anxiety, hyperacusis, depression, insomnia, and other symptoms they may experience in association with it.

Pros: More effective than medications for relieving stress-related conditions that often trigger or worsen tinnitus symptoms such as depression and anxiety. CBT can provide long-lasting relief from this condition if you practice the techniques regularly over time, so they become automatic habits in dealing with your thoughts and response to them.

Cons: Cognitive behavioral therapy requires that you participate actively in it, such as by practicing relaxation techniques, changing the way you think about your symptoms, recording your symptoms, and following through with various strategies that are suggested to you.

Medications

Certain medications are believed to help reduce tinnitus symptoms in some people. These include antidepressants that affect serotonin levels, anti-seizure drugs, steroids, and blood pressure medications.

Pros: These may be used to treat the symptoms associated with Tinnitus, including anxiety, depression, insomnia, and stress.

They are also relatively inexpensive.

Cons: Some people do not get good results from taking medication to treat their Tinnitus. In addition, those who take medications may have side effects such as increased fatigue and blurred vision.

Lifestyle Changes

Making these changes is often referred to as "tinnitus retraining therapy," which you can learn more about in the next chapter.

Pros: These changes often reduce stress levels, which is helpful if This common trigger factor causes tinnitus. It is also relatively inexpensive and can provide long-term relief from this condition in most people.

Cons: Requires that you practice these changes consistently over time, so they become effective methods of dealing with your tinnitus symptoms.

Ear canal inserts

These are also called hearing aids. These devices deliver sound directly into the ear(s) through a small earpiece inserted in the ear canal. The best part about them is that you can use them even if you have not lost your hearing. The key is to equip them with tinnitus-masking features to drown out internal noise and offer relief. It is a popular treatment option often coupled with other hearing loss treatment options.

These devices work by providing relief from subjective noises such as hissing and buzzing while allowing people to hear what goes on around them. The wearer must often select the frequency and level of sound delivered via this form.

Pros: Produce sounds that cover up the annoying and bothersome sounds associated with Tinnitus. They can also be effective means of reducing stress and providing relief from this condition when compared to medications and CBT in some cases.

Cons: When you wear them, people around you may not be able to hear what you are listening to if they may be important for you, such as a radio or television show. In addition, ear canal inserts may become uncomfortable after wearing them for long periods, such as while sleeping.

Tinnitus Retraining Therapy (TRT)

TRT is a treatment option that couples counseling with sound therapy, both of which are based on the neurophysiological model of the condition. The main aim of using TRT is to leverage the brain's natural abilities to habituate signals and filter out any noise at the subconscious level to prevent it from getting to the conscious level.

The best part about habituation is that it doesn't require conscious effort. Typically, humans habituate such noises as those coming from computer fans, air conditioners, or rains because they are non-important; hence the brain does not register them as loud.

With this therapy, a tinnitus patient must play some kind of neutral sounds everywhere they go by wearing in-the-ear sound generators. They are also given counseling. This treatment option takes 12-24 months to correct the problem completely.

Pros: This form of treatment is considered to be the one with the highest success rate for improving and often completely relieving the bothersome and sometimes painful symptoms associated with chronic Tinnitus in most cases. TRT enables you to improve your quality of life by giving you greater control over when and for how long your symptoms occur and allowing you to reduce stress levels associated with them, such as by silencing the ringing in your ears when you want them to. Later chapters in this guide will discuss this a bit more.

Cons: This treatment option is often done for a year or two, which requires that you spend time with a qualified tinnitus specialist who can help guide you through it successfully.

PREVENTING TINNITUS

There is no known method for preventing this condition from developing at present. Nevertheless, you can take some steps to reduce your likelihood of developing tinnitus if you are worried about experiencing it due to something that may trigger it, such as an ear injury or exposure to loud noise. These include:

Take breaks from loud noises if possible, and always wear ear protection if you know that your work or other activities may lead to a greater risk of experiencing tinnitus symptoms.

Limit the amount of time you spend listening to loud noises such as rock concerts, music at high volume levels, and even television shows. In addition, try to turn down the volume on electronic devices such as computer monitors, stereos, and televisions before you reach a point where it becomes uncomfortable.

One of the most important things to remember about tinnitus is that if you continue to expose yourself to loud noise, your chances of developing this condition will be greater. At the same time, take steps to reduce these risks by maintaining a safe listening volume level whenever you need to be around loud noise.

Other ways to prevent tinnitus are exercising, eating healthily, drinking plenty of water, getting enough sleep, learning how to relax your mind and body, reducing stress levels as much as possible, and practicing mindfulness techniques.

Of course, it is not always possible to control the factors that may increase your likelihood of developing tinnitus. The good news is that by learning more about its symptoms and using available and effective treatments, you can reduce the impact this condition has on your quality of life. It will also help you remain calm if it does develop, which is an important part of remaining in control of your symptoms.

Often, people ask whether earplugs can cause tinnitus. The truth is that earplugs cannot cause tinnitus. However, they have been shown to cause tinnitus-like symptoms. Traditional earplugs are made from pliable materials that can be inserted into the ear to cancel out any noise from the external environment. They are often used by people who wish to fall asleep or need to protect their ears from noisy surroundings.

According to the University of Manchester researchers, when earplugs are worn by people who don't have tinnitus, they experience a form of "hearing loss" produced by phantom buzzing or ringing sounds in the ear; but dissipates once the earplugs are taken off.

On the other hand, when tinnitus patients wear these earplugs, they exaggerate the buzzing or ringing sounds in the ears by blocking all outside noises, which, in turn, strengthens the earplugs' internal ringing sound intended to drown out in the first place. This way, the symptoms are perceived to have worsened. You must understand that this is not permanent. As soon as you take off the earplugs, the exaggerated ringing sound will disappear.

Therefore, if you suffer from tinnitus, you must take extra care to protect your hearing. Ask yourself, what triggers my tinnitus? Is it loud due to music, traffic, or construction work? Whatever is triggering your tinnitus, note that using noise-canceling plugs goes a long way in relieving the symptoms and protecting your ear from further damage.

To prevent tinnitus, you can choose to use high-fidelity earplugs, typically used by musicians, to protect your hearing without necessarily blocking out all sounds from your environment. What I love most about these earplugs is that they have acoustic filters that allow you to fine-tune sound frequency, prevent tinnitus triggers, and reduce the symptoms by significantly lowering the sound levels.

ALL ABOUT TINNITUS RETRAINING THERAPY

Tinnitus retraining therapy, or TRT, is an innovative treatment option for chronic tinnitus sufferers developed by Dr. Pawel Jastreboff of Emory University in Atlanta, Georgia, during the early 1990s who first published his ideas and findings of this form of treatment. His research showed that chronic Tinnitus is caused not just by hearing loss but also by how we perceive these bothersome sounds.

To explain further, our brains learn to link some external stimuli, such as tinnitus, to a physiological irritation or injury. In the case of this condition, sufferers experience these bothersome sounds in their ears even though no such sound is present in reality.

By learning to ignore tinnitus symptoms, TRT enables people who are affected by chronic tinnitus to re-establish the link between these symptoms and their actual cause, which is psychological. This form of treatment does not cure tinnitus but simply enables sufferers to modify how they perceive this condition so that it does not hurt their mental well-being or interfere with doing what needs to be done each day.

TRT involves three basic steps, which are:

- **Habituation**: This step will enable you to learn how best to tune out the constant ringing, hissing, or other noises associated with chronic Tinnitus so that they no longer have an impact on your life. You will do this by wearing noise generators to cancel out the bothersome noises associated with this condition. Some noise generators are small enough to fit inside the ear canal, while others are larger devices that can be worn in or behind your ears. You can find a noise generator by doing an online search for "tinnitus masking devices."

• **Identification**: This step involves learning how to identify the cause of Tinnitus. You will know when it is safe for you to use sound generators and other treatment tools so they do not interfere with what you need to get done each day. You also learn how to establish control over this condition by using customized sound therapies, relaxation techniques, and various drugs or medicines used for stress relief or sleep enhancement if needed.

• **Control**: The final step in TRT enables chronic tinnitus sufferers to achieve a greater degree of control over their condition by retraining their brains into responding differently whenever these bothersome sounds occur in the future.

HOW TO GET STARTED WITH TRT

T innitus retraining therapy is one of the advances in tinnitus research that has made it possible for people to live and cope with the condition. With TRT, you learn to cope with tinnitus on both conscious and subconscious levels.

Ideally, the therapy aims to "retrain" the main internal systems involved, which are the auditory, limbic, and autonomic nervous systems. Following that order, these systems deal with hearing, emotions, and the flight or fight response. Retraining these internal systems may change the way they receive, process, and interpret sound. This may also teach these systems to stop creating the same buzzing or ringing sounds. TRT also attempts to understand why you hear these sounds to properly address them.

Usually, Tinnitus Retraining Therapy lasts for about 12-24 months. The therapy has 3 main goals that must be met to assure its effectiveness:

• **Educate regarding the condition.** This is important because it will help the patient understand that what they're experiencing is because of tinnitus—whether it's the primary cause or a complication. Because this condition affects not only their auditory senses but also their emotional and mental state, the patient must be made to understand clearly how tinnitus affects them wholly.

This is also why it's important to seek the help and assistance of a specialist in doing this therapy. Being able to receive the proper help from an expert or specialist will greatly benefit the patient.

● **Start habituation of tinnitus.** This is when retraining of the involved internal systems happens. Habituation refers to the condition where the subject is made to become habituated or accustomed to something by doing an action or a stimulus repeatedly.

To explain how it works, it's similar to this: for example, you live near the main road where there's heavy traffic or by the beach, you probably noticed the noise when you first moved in. However, as time passes, you get used to the familiar noise around you. Somehow, you become desensitized by it.

Another similar scenario is when you're trying to review or read something. When you start, you may still be sensitive to the noise or to what's happening around you. However, when you start to focus more on what you're doing or reading, the noise also tends to bother or affect you less, and you tend to get used to it until it doesn't bother you anymore.

That's how habituation works. It kind of tells your systems that tinnitus or the noise you hear isn't important and can and must be ignored.

● **Neutralize negative reaction**

Along with habituation, a tinnitus patient must also be "retrained" to think that the noise isn't something to react negatively to—emotionally, physiologically, and psychologically.

Usually, these reactions that you express towards tinnitus are considered obstacles that hinder the habituation from naturally occurring. It's a difficult process and not something that promises instant relief. It will take time, also this will greatly require patience, discipline, and determination.

In the article "The Tinnitus Retraining Therapy Trial (TRTT): study protocol for a randomized controlled trial" by the Tinnitus Retraining Therapy Trial Research Group, they also noted a couple more primary subgoals of TRT, which are:

- habituation of tinnitus-evoked negative reaction

- habituation of perception

The first one aims to recognize and understand how a patient reacts to tinnitus. Some of the negative tinnitus-related reactions include feeling annoyed, anxious, or panicked. Because patients don't usually know they have tinnitus and what they're hearing is something that they can learn to ignore, they feel frustrated. The second one now focuses on making the patient aware of tinnitus and how they can tune this out, which may eventually help the patient be more conscious of the symptoms as well as start to neutralize the patient's reaction towards it.

During the habituation phases, sound therapy is also done. Remember the scenario described in the previous pages? When you get used to the noise, you eventually learn to ignore them until they no longer affect you. It's the same with sound therapy.

Managing tinnitus at home

After understanding how tinnitus retraining therapy works, it's time to consult your doctor or a specialist if this is something you want to try. Look for an expert or ask your doctor for a recommendation on where to consult with an auditory specialist.

You can also try out simple steps to help with your therapy. There are tinnitus apps that you can use to help you with managing this condition. In a user survey published by the National Library for Medicine called "Mobile Apps for Management of Tinnitus: Users' Survey, Quality Assessment, and Content Analysis," the researchers listed mobile apps and narrowed them down to specific categories based on uses, quality, and content. The research had 643 respondents,

There were 120 respondents out of the 643 who listed 55 apps they have used for tinnitus management. Based on the research, 14 of these apps were specifically developed for tinnitus, either to distract or provide relief from it.

Further categorization is as follows:

Apps with implemented management programs specifically for tinnitus:

- iTinnitus
- Tinnitus Balance
- Tinnitus Management
- Widex Zen

Apps that use sound aiming to distract or give relief from tinnitus:

- Sound Relief
- Tinnitus Therapy Lite
- Tinnitus Therapy Tunes

Apps that have combination exercises for sound and relaxation:

- Beltone Tinnitus Calmer
- ReSound Relief

Other apps you may want to check out:

- Starkey Relax - provides resource materials for the users along with sound therapy exercises
- Tinnitus Measurer - aims to measure the pitch of tinnitus
- Overcome Tinnitus - uses hypnosis

The rest of the apps in the study mostly fell under the category of providing relaxation, concentration, etc. without explicitly mentioning tinnitus as one of their targeted uses.

CONCLUSION

It is no secret that living with tinnitus can be challenging. Most people experience the temporary signs of Tinnitus at some point in their life, perhaps due to ear infections or exposure to loud noise, among other causes. Struggling with tinnitus symptoms every day can be downright depressing, hence why finding treatment options that offer relief is key.

You can gain a personalized treatment plan by choosing to work closely with hearing professionals. This way, they can tailor a plan that suits your specific hearing needs. Realize that even moderate levels of Tinnitus have been known to affect one's ability to work and socialize. It often triggers anxiety, making it hard to fall asleep, hence worsening anxiety.

The key to a successful recovery is using strategies that will break the vicious cycle, which by the way, is often a hard nut to crack!

The good news is that there is HOPE.

By following the treatment options, we have discussed in this article, you can effectively lower your response to noise stimulus with repeated exposure and get to a point where Tinnitus is no longer bothersome. The key is to catch yourself checking in with the noise. Recognize that just like raindrops pounding on a roof; the intensity will go down once you train your brain to filter it out as unimportant.

Learn to remind yourself that this too will pass continually. The moment you start to experience the ringing sound in your ear, immediately pick a coping tool to use before you get back to your routine. You will realize that these coping tools will gradually help you mask the tinnitus sounds and allow you to relax both physically and mentally.

So, what are you still waiting for?

It's time to break the vicious cycle of tinnitus and live your life to the fullest!

REFERENCES

A step-by-step guide to tinnitus sound therapy | decibel hearing services | blog. (n.d.). Https://Decibelhearing.Com/. Retrieved November 26, 2022, from https://decibelhearing.com/a-step-by-step-guide-to-tinnitus-sound-therapy/.

Chari, D. A., & Limb, C. J. (2018). Tinnitus. Medical Clinics, 102(6), 1081-1093.

FAAA, D. J. P., Au D. (2020, April 28). Does tinnitus retraining therapy work? Sound Relief Hearing Center. https://www.soundrelief.com/does-tinnitus-retraining-therapy-work/.

Gold, S. L., Formby, C., & Scherer, R. W. (2021). The tinnitus retraining therapy counseling protocol is implemented in the Tinnitus Retraining Therapy Trial. American journal of audiology, 30(1), 1-15.

Jastreboff, P. J. (2011). Tinnitus retraining therapy. Textbook of Tinnitus, 575-596.

Jastreboff, P. J., & Jastreboff, M. M. (2006). Tinnitus retraining therapy: a different view on Tinnitus. Orl, 68(1), 23-30.

Phillips, J. S., & McFerran, D. (2010). Tinnitus retraining therapy (TRT) for Tinnitus. Cochrane database of systematic reviews, (3).

Scherer, R. W., Formby, C., & Tinnitus Retraining Therapy Trial Research Group. (2019). A randomized clinical trial is the effect of tinnitus retraining therapy vs. standard of care on tinnitus-related quality of life. JAMA Otolaryngology–Head & Neck

Surgery, 145(7), 597-608.

Sedley, W. (2019). Tinnitus: does gain explain? Neuroscience, 407, 213-228.

Sereda, M., Smith, S., Newton, K., & Stockdale, D. (2019). Mobile apps for management of tinnitus: Users' survey, quality assessment, and content analysis. JMIR MHealth and UHealth, 7(1), e10353. https://doi.org/10.2196/10353.

Sereda, M., Xia, J., El Refaie, A., Hall, D. A., & Hoare, D. J. (2018). Sound therapy (using amplification devices and/or sound generators) for Tinnitus. Cochrane Database of Systematic Reviews, (12).

Tinnitus habituation: How to tune out the ringing in your ears. (n.d.). Healthy Hearing. Retrieved November 26, 2022, from https://www.healthyhearing.com/report/52940-Tinnitus-habituation-how-to-tune-out-the-ringing-in-your-ears.

Tinnitus Retraining Therapy Trial Research Group, Scherer, R. W., Formby, C., Gold, S., Erdman, S., Rodhe, C., Carlson, M., Shade, D., Tucker, M., Sensinger, L. M., Hughes, G., Conley, G. S., Downey, N., Eades, C., Jylkka, M., Haber-Perez, A., Harper, C., Russell, S. K., Sierra-Irizarry, B., & Sullivan, M. (2014). The Tinnitus Retraining Therapy Trial (Trtt): Study protocol for a randomized controlled trial. Trials, 15(1), 396. https://doi.org/10.1186/1745-6215-15-396

Tinnitus. Org | trt excercises. (n.d.). Retrieved November 26, 2022, from https://tinnitus.org/trt-excercises/.

Wang, H., Tang, D., Wu, Y., Zhou, L., & Sun, S. (2020). The state of the art of sound therapy for subjective Tinnitus in adults. Therapeutic Advances in Chronic Disease, 11, 2040622320956426.

Printed in Great Britain
by Amazon

27665537R10020